From
Diagnosis
To
MANAGEMENT

A Guide for People Over 50 with Type 2 Diabetes

Trinette Stanford
MSN, FNP-C, CDCES, MBA

Printed in the United States of America

ISBN: 9798388965509

Totally About Diabetes, LLC
Abbeville, AL 36310
TotallyAboutDiabetes.com
info@totallyaboutdiabetes.com

This book is a labor of love. My heart's desire is to help people that have type 2 diabetes or prediabetes to have the skills and tools to manage their condition. Hopefully the message will resonate with someone and change their life.

Thank You...

for purchasing this book. As my gift to you, please visit
TotallyAboutDiabetes.com/ResourceGuide

Also, don't forget to leave a review on Amazon.

Table of Contents

Introduction

Why I chose to write this book? I have heard so many people say, just move more and eat less and you will lose weight and get rid of diabetes. Unfortunately, that advice does not work for many people. Granted some people do develop type 2 diabetes after gaining weight but guess what? There are many people who are morbidly obese, who don't have diabetes. There are many people of "normal weight" with type 2 diabetes. Go figure. You cannot make assumptions by just looking at people.

There are people who have embraced lifestyle behavior change – exercise, lose weight, etc. and still have diabetes.

Now understand, I am not telling people not to lose weight. Obesity causes so many other health problems, so it does help to improve health by losing weight. But this book is a guide for healthier living. The title says diabetes, but these same habits and steps listed will help people with all types of chronic health problems such as heart disease, kidney disease, and chronic lung problems.

This book is from the perspective of an over 50-year-old (over 60) woman, post-menopausal, and with hypertension. I have been a nurse for over 40 years, a family nurse practitioner for over 30 years, and a diabetes educator for over 25 years. I have treated many people with diabetes, mostly type 2. Some things I have learned over the years is:

- Everybody's body is different.

- Nothing should be off limits, but they must learn how to limit themselves.

- In this book, I will avoid using the word diet when discussing a meal plan. I will focus on the way of eating.

- I will not stress or harp on weight in this book. It is best to manage our weight for good health. There are many circumstances, especially among women over the age of 50, that have struggled with weight. In this book, the focus is on healthy living, which includes eating the right foods. Other habits that promote health are highlighted in the following pages.

- The most successful diabetes management plan is personal and individualized. I want to encourage the reader to set their own goals. After setting their goals, then develop a plan that will get them to their goal.

As a mature nurse, I have learned to listen to people. One of my first doctor employers told me that if you let people talk, they will eventually tell you what is wrong with them. That has proven true over the years. Successful diabetes management is:

- Shared decision making – between the provider and the client

- Client-centered, client-focused care – this is the obligation of the provider

Shared decision-making is finding out what the client is willing to do, what changes they are willing to make, and making a plan using that information. Client-centered care is planning where the client is the focus, but we, the client and provider, desire the same outcome.

The goal of diabetes management is to manage and control diabetes, prevent complications, and avoid hospitalizations. The problem with type 2 diabetes is it does not hurt until something serious has occurred. Type 2 diabetes is one of those chronic diseases that occurs without you being aware. There is not a time when you can point to say that is when it started. By the time people are diagnosed with diabetes, it can be present for 6 – 10 years. That is why it is important for you to have a primary care provider you can trust and talk to.

Providing information on type 2 diabetes to people over the age of 50 can be particularly helpful, as this population is at a higher risk of developing the condition.

We will review those risk factors later in the book. Let's review what diabetes is and the different types.

Disclaimer: This content is for educational purposes only. Do not use the content of this book as a substitute for direct medical or clinical advice from your doctor or other qualified clinicians.

Chapter 1: Types of Diabetes

There are multiple types of diabetes, but these are the most common ones. Terms to understand glucose is blood sugar. Pancreas is the organ that produces insulin.

Type 1 – this is an autoimmune condition where the pancreas has stopped producing insulin. It used to be called juvenile diabetes because children usually developed it. But Type 1 can occur at any age. Any injury or insult to the pancreas can cause it to shut down. A tumor or medication can be responsible. People with type 1 diabetes must receive insulin injections to live. Symptoms include significant weight loss because the body is not able to use blood sugar, so it uses body mass to feed itself. Increased urination because of high blood sugar, increased thirst because of dehydration from increased urination. One tell-tale sign is a fruity odor to the breath (acetone). Without medical attention, the client starts to have drowsiness and lethargy that can lead to an unconscious state. The body has increased ketones which can be deadly if not hospitalized. This is not the same ketone condition that occurs with a ketogenic diet.

Type 2 – this is a chronic condition where the body either does not produce enough insulin for the body to operate efficiently or insulin resistance occurs. Insulin resistance is when the pancreas produces insulin, but it cannot get into the cells to join with the glucose to break the glucose down. In insulin resistance, the body senses that the glucose is high, so the body produces more insulin, but it is blocked from the glucose. So, you end up with high blood sugar and high insulin levels. These reactions are subtle. What you may notice is weight gain, especially around the midsection. Increased insulin leads to increased hunger. By the way, insulin is a fat-storing hormone. Other symptoms are increased urination because of the high glucose and increased thirst due to the increased urination. This causes dehydration. Some may experience some weight loss due to excessive urination. The urine contains a large amount of glucose. You are peeing out your calories. Some other symptoms that may occur are numbness or tingling of feet.

Gestational diabetes – this type of diabetes is diagnosed during pregnancy. It usually goes away after delivery, but the danger is the mother can develop type 2 diabetes later in life. The danger of gestational diabetes is that the baby can be excessively large. The way it is diagnosed, the mother has a glucose tolerance test (GTT), usually at six months of pregnancy. If the mother is diagnosed with gestational diabetes, they usually are placed on insulin because it is the only medicine that can cross the placenta and get to the baby. That way, the mother and the baby are treated. Of course, the mother is placed on a special diet to go along with the medication treatment.

Mature onset diabetes in the young (MODY) – this is a type 2 diabetes that occurs in very young children. It is different from type 1 diabetes because the body can still produce insulin, but the body is unable to use it properly. This type of diabetes will require referral to an endocrinologist.

Latent autoimmune diabetes in adults (LADA) – this is a type 1 diabetes that occurs in adults, but it is a subtle and slow onset. Usually, these people are treated as type 2 initially but find they are not responding to therapy. Instead of improving, their condition worsens. This type requires specialist intervention (endocrinologist) and specialized testing. There are hormones and antibodies that need to be evaluated for accurate diagnosis. LADA clients must be on insulin for treatment. Unfortunately, they generally have wide swings and extreme lows with significant highs before they can be placed on the correct regimen.

That is why it is important that you have a primary care provider that is aware of the different types of diabetes and how to treat it. It can be a matter of life and death.

The focus of this book is on type 2 diabetes and its related conditions. Next, we will discuss the diabetes spectrum. There is a linear progression that takes place, and the sooner the symptoms are recognized, the sooner intervention can be started.

Chapter 2: The Diabetes Spectrum

Diabetes is a progressive disease. Type 2 diabetes just doesn't appear overnight. It is a chronic disease that usually takes years to develop. The underlying cause of the process can be multifaceted. Genetics and family history are some of the main causes. Your family line has a history of type 2 diabetes. It may be a genetic defect or a family history of lifestyle habits. Unhealthy foods and meal habits are passed down from generation to generation. Think about it. What did your family drink when you were growing up? I know my family lived on Kool-Aid. Back then, it came in small packs, and you had to add sugar. Imagine how much sugar we consume just by drinking Kool-Aid. Sodas or pop was a treat when I was growing up, just like fast food places. That was a once-a-month trip to Burger King. But I did grow up on the standard American diet. A meat, a starch, and a vegetable for dinner. Usually, sandwiches for lunch – processed meat and cheese on white bread. Back then, Wonder bread was the go-to. When I had children, the same pattern continued. The only difference was I made a lot of casseroles because they were quick and easy and had leftovers. Kool-Aid was the go-to again.

A sedentary lifestyle is another habit that can be passed down through the generations. So, think about your childhood and adulthood. Do you notice a pattern? Well, this pattern sets the stage for the Diabetes Spectrum.

The first part of the spectrum is a metabolic syndrome where high blood pressure develops, and cholesterol issues may occur. This step is subtle and may not be realized until you get your blood pressure checked at a provider visit. There may be a hint of cholesterol issues in the lab work but nothing serious. They may tell you that LDL is a little high and HDL is a little low. They may recommend you exercise or move about more.

The next step is insulin resistance. Again, this step is basically asymptomatic, but there are some subtle changes. You may notice some weight gain, especially around the midsection. What is happening behind the scenes is muscles, fat, and the liver don't respond to the insulin released from the pancreas. The insulin is unable to metabolize the glucose. The glucose is supposed to get into the muscle cells for nourish-ment. The insulin is unable to get to the glucose. So the glucose ends up being stored as fat in the body and the liver. Insulin is a hormone secreted by the pancreas to help break down glucose in the body. The main problem with insulin resistance is weight gain. Lab work may or may not show some slight abnormalities but nothing serious. As time progresses and no lifestyle changes take place, then the next step occurs.

Prediabetes has gained attention in the last few years as the precursor to type 2 diabetes. Programs have been developed to prevent type 2 diabetes by intervening at the prediabetes stage. One in three adults in the US had prediabetes. The real danger is 8 out of 10 are unaware that they have prediabetes. Prediabetes is identified with fasting blood sugar greater than 110 and less than 126 on two separate occasions. The A1C is greater than 5.5 and less than 6.5. The risk factors for prediabetes are:

- Overweight or obese
- Older than 45 years old
- Family history of type 2 diabetes
- Little physical activity
- History of gestational diabetes

Those who are at higher risk are African – Americans, Hispanics, American Indians, Pacific Islanders, and Asian- Americans.

The seriousness of prediabetes is the high risk of heart attack and stroke. Women at childbirth age experience PCOS – polycystic ovarian syndrome. This condition interferes with fertility in women. But if you look at the spectrum in the earlier stages, there may have been a chance to avoid the prediabetes stage. Early identification and early intervention can prevent long-term problems and complications.

The next stage that develops if no intervention is successful at prediabetes is type 2 diabetes. Early stages of type 2 diabetes being identified by fasting glucose greater than 126 on two different occasions, A1C greater than 6.5, or abnormal glucose tolerance test (GTT) greater than 200 at any stage. This is the stage where aggressive lifestyle changes are recommended. Nutrition or dietician referral may be given, as well as diabetes education classes may be encouraged. Depending on lab values, follow-up visits may be 3-6 months. If no improvement has occurred, medication may be ordered. Many people are resistant to starting on medications, but sometimes medications are needed to get you back on the right track.

When type 2 diabetes is diagnosed, hopefully, it will be in the early stages.

Chapter 3: A.V.O.I.D. Complications

Complications occur in the later stages of type 2 diabetes. The goal of therapy is to A.V.O.I.D. complications. Notice how to avoid is printed out. It is an acronym to show what complications can occur if diabetes is not controlled.

A – Amputation. This is one of the most feared and visible complications that can occur. Amputation is life-altering and can lead to disability. The amputation is a result of tissue damage due to infection or impaired circulation. It can affect the toe(s), foot, and leg. It all depends on where the damage is. To avoid this complication, one must be vigilant in their care. Make sure blood sugars are controlled and avoid injury to feet. Wearing shoes is always an easy way to protect your feet from blunt force trauma or injury. Inspect your feet every day. Look at the bottom of your feet and between your toes daily. If you're not mobile or flexible enough, have someone else inspect your feet or use a mirror to look. We will go into further detail about foot care in a later chapter.

V - Vascular. Vascular has to do with circulation throughout the body. Uncontrolled diabetes can cause elevated cholesterol, which can lead to blockages in different parts of the body. Vascular comprises 2 parts, microvascular, which means small vessels, and macrovascular, which means large vessels. The organs affected are the heart and brain. Bad circulation to the heart can lead to a heart attack, and impaired circulation to the brain can lead to a stroke. Again, we are looking at life–altering complications. A heart attack weakens and damages the heart muscle. This damage can affect how you are able to function every day. It can affect your energy and ability to operate. A stroke affects part of the brain. It all depends on the location and what part of the body is affected. There may be some weakness or impairment of the legs and arms. Speech and thought processes may also be affected. So, it is vitally important to keep those vessels open.

O – Ocular. This refers to the eyes. Remember we spoke about microvascular damage in the vascular area? Well, the eyes receive blood supply from the microvascular system. Uncontrolled diabetes affects the vessels by causing bleeding behind the eye. This condition is called retinopathy. Untreated retinopathy can cause vision loss and progress to blindness. Like all chronic diseases, there are no noticeable symptoms in the beginning. That is why routine dilated eye exams are necessary to detect these problems. Other problems that can occur are increased pressure leading to glaucoma or cataract formation. These are treatable conditions that are preventable with diligent care and routine exams.

I – Impotence. This is a complication caused by impaired circulation to the genital and pelvic area. This complication affects men and women. It is more noticeable in men having erectile dysfunction. But women lose sensation in their clitoris and vaginal area. Those blood vessels are essential to continue with sexual health and well-being.

D – Dialysis. This is a dreaded complication. Dialysis occurs with kidney or renal failure. This is a chronic problem; just like type 2 diabetes, kidney failure does not occur overnight. Kidney disease occurs in stages. Chronic kidney disease, just like other chronic problems, is unnoticeable as it occurs. It is only detected through lab work. That is why it is important to have regular visits with labs. I recommend that you get copies of your labs to compare them. One set of labs is like a snapshot, and it is a record of what is going on at that period of time. When you compare them, any change can be detected to see what the trends are. For instance, kidney function tests are creatinine, BUN, eGFR, and albumin. The eGFR shows the kidney filter property and albumin shows kidney damage. How have the tests been? Are they staying within the same range, or are the creatinine, BUN, and albumin rising? Is the eGFR declining? If so, this is a sign of kidney function decline. Kidney disease is staged according to eGFR, and interventions can be done to prevent or slow down the decline of the kidney condition.

Chapter 4: Speaking of Labs

It's important to pay attention to other labs. I'm going to try to keep this understandable. Different lab companies set different ranges. Please consult with your provider or his representative to discuss your case. It is important you can discuss and understand your laboratory values. Comparing your last labs with your present labs will help to detect any trends or changes that can point to potential problems.

This is just an overview to provide some foundation of understanding. I'm not going to list every single element, just the pertinent ones that pertain to diabetes.

CMP or Comprehensive Metabolic Profile
This group of tests look at the following:

- Glucose – this is your blood sugar at the time your blood was drawn

- Potassium – this is an element essential for heart and muscle health.

- BUN, creatinine, eGFR, albumin – these show the condition of your kidneys.

- Total protein, alkaline phosphatase (ALP), alanine transaminase (ALT), aspartate aminotransferase (AST) – these are related to the health of your liver

- Hemoglobin A1C – a test that shows an average of blood sugar over the last three months. The results of this test may not be accurate in pregnancy, anemia (sickle cell or Thalassemia), recent trauma, or blood transfusion.

- Lipid panel
  - Cholesterol – This is an overall result of your cholesterol.

  - Triglycerides – circulating fats within the bloodstream. When our bodies are not able to use all the calories we eat, the excess calories are stored in triglycerides.

  - HDL – considered the "good" cholesterol. This protein carries the LDL particles to the liver to be flushed out from the body.

  - LDL – considered bad cholesterol. LDL carries cholesterol to the cells and the liver. Too much LDL causes blockages in the arteries.

To get the most accurate lab results, it is best to do them fasting. The fast is generally more than 8 hours. A1C can be done non-fasting.

- Vitamin D – is not part of routine labs. It must be ordered separately. Vitamin D is an essential vitamin to help with blood sugar control. It is also beneficial in slowing the growth of cancer cells, reduce infection and inflammation. You need vitamin D to maintain healthy bones and a healthy heart.

- CBC – complete blood count. It may or may not be included in standard labs.

  - WBC – white blood count. The total number of white blood cells. Elevation may be related to infection or some disease.

  - RBC – red blood count. The total number of red blood cells. This group of tests is used to diagnose anemia.

  - Platelet count – these are vital for clotting. They prevent and stop bleeding.

Chapter 5: Speak English, Please!

This chapter will discuss how to manage blood sugar levels and explain common terminology.

Hyperglycemia – this means high blood sugar, generally higher than 200. This can be dangerous if it is greater than 250 most of the time. Another term is **blood sugar spikes** – this means the blood sugar goes extremely high very fast. Occasional highs are acceptable, but they should not be a common everyday occurrence. This usually happens after eating or drinking a large amount of simple carbohydrates without any protein or fat to balance it. The symptoms are:

- Extreme drowsiness
- Excessive thirst
- Increased urination

The best way to lower blood sugar quickly and safely is by drinking 16 – 24 ounces of water. This will dilute the sugar, and then go for a walk. Check your blood sugar first. If it's around 200, go for a 10 -15-minute walk. Walking will burn off that extra sugar by driving it to the muscles in the legs and thighs. If you are unable to go for a walk outdoors, march in place and do some mild squats. Act like you're sitting in a chair and then stand up. This movement activates the thighs and buttock (glute) muscles.

Your target is to get your sugar around 100.

Hypoglycemia – this means low blood sugar. Symptoms of hypoglycemia are:
- Fast heartbeat
- Shakiness
- Sweating
- Confusion
- Irritability
- Dizziness

Low blood sugars can be life–threatening. Untreated hypoglycemia, especially very low readings, can lead to unconsciousness and seizures. This is the life-threatening part. The goal of therapy is to raise the blood sugar to more than 80 as fast as possible. Steps for treating hypoglycemia is the rule of 15:

- Check your blood sugar.

- Less than 70 (60 – 70). The quick sugar fix plan. **15** Grams of simple carbohydrates for treatment. That would be one of the following options: 4 ounces of orange juice, apple juice, regular pop, or soda; one tablespoon of sugar or 5 Lifesavers, or other hard candies. There are glucose tablets available, too. The usual dose is four tablets to raise blood sugar. Don't use low-sugar or diet products to treat hypoglycemia. Avoid using chocolate to raise blood sugar because the fat in the chocolate will slow down the absorption of the sugar.

- Wait **15** minutes, and then recheck your blood sugar. If it's higher than 80 and close to mealtime, eat your meal. If not at mealtime, eat a snack of complex carbohydrates and protein. Such as ½ sandwich of whole grain bread and meat, tuna, nut butter, or something similar. A hard-boiled egg is a good snack, too. You want to eat to avoid your blood sugar dropping again after it uses the quick sugar fix.

- If your **blood sugar is less than 50**, immediate attention is needed. You will need 30 grams of carbohydrates to raise your blood sugar to a normal level. Eight ounces of regular soda, orange, or apple juice, or two tablespoons of sugar in 4 ounces of water. Glucagon injection gives a great response for super low readings. Glucagon is an injection of a hormone that causes a fast release of glucose by the liver. If glucagon is not available, use a liquid form of simple sugar like jelly or honey. Placing sugar substances under the tongue is absorbed faster.

You will see an immediate response to the added sugar. Remember, it is still important to eat a meal or a snack after the treatment to keep the blood sugars up.

Hemoglobin A1C – this is the routine blood test done on people with diabetes, usually every three months. This test is an average of your blood sugars. The normal rate for people without diabetes is less than 5.3%. For people with diabetes, the goal is 6.5 – 7%. For high-risk people- with multiple illnesses, frail, or older than 75, an A1C of 8.0% is acceptable. The reason for the difference is that low A1C has an increased risk of many hypoglycemic or low blood sugar episodes. It is better for high-risk people to run a little higher than too low. The A1C does not provide accurate readings for people with sickle cell or other anemias, or if one has had a recent transfusion or injury.

Glucometer – A meter used to check blood sugar. Using the meter requires finger sticks and the use of strips. The strips are the most expensive part of this device. You must be careful of the storage of the meter and strips. Do not keep them in the car for long periods of time. Temperature changes can damage the strips. Also, check the expiration date. Out-of-date strips can give you false readings.

CGM Continuous Glucose Meter – is a newer technology that uses a sensor that is placed on an area that has padding and stays flat. The beauty of the CGM, blood sugar readings can be done by looking at the transmitter or phone. There are different CGMs on the market and each has its own method of operation. The CGM is ideal for people who must do multiple checks a day, are on insulin, or have problems handling the strips. The use of CGM helps the user keep blood sugars in control because they are aware of their readings. You will be able to see how certain foods affect your blood sugars.

Chapter 6: Five Pillars of Healthy Living

There are five concepts that I use in teaching about healthy living to people with diabetes and other chronic diseases.

- Mindset
- Healthy Nutrition
- Exercise
- Effective Sleep
- Stress Management

MINDSET

Mindset is the 1st pillar of healthy living. What's your viewpoint? Is the glass always half empty or half full?

This is the time a decision is made for your future. It is time to look inward.

- Mindfulness
- Awareness
- Evaluate your body and mind.

This keeps us anchored or grounded. Making these considerations keeps us in the present. If you think it, you can achieve it. The emotional/mental action precedes the physical response.

Harness your mind!

Willpower and discipline are an exercise of the mind. When you strengthen your mind, your thought processes help bring your body and actions into line. Breathing exercises and meditation practice help to bring you back into the present. When you take time to think and process you will avoid getting caught up in the moment. Take time to acknowledge and admit the situation. This acknowledgment will decrease distress and increase your control. Celebrate small victories, they lead to bigger rewards.

Willpower is for right now. Exercise is repeated successful uses of willpower that will lead to the habit of self-discipline.

Healthy Thoughts to Use Every Day:
- Desire to do better.
- Be mindful of what you eat.
- Be mindful of how you move.
- Move more.
- Sleep better.
- Decrease stress.

Small steps of pleasure will assist in propelling you forward to a rewarding healthy life.

1. Meditation/prayer – to help set your intention for the day.
2. Plan out daily activities – put your intentions into a plan.
3. Plan meals for the day
4. Interact and consult with others – Work with accountability partners to help keep you on track

HEALTHY NUTRITION

Healthy nutrition is the 2nd pillar of healthy living. Let's face it, your circumstances changed when you were diagnosed with diabetes/prediabetes. Now, what are you going to do about it? Remember, back in the mindset, you have decided that you desire to do better. Let's put it into action.

You've heard the saying, "You are what you eat"? However, Tracy Harrison from the School of Functional Medicine says it best, "You are what you eat, chew, swallow, digest, and absorb."

What you eat makes up about 75% of your health journey. It is time to set the intention to start eating healthy. Here are five steps to take:

1. Start slow – Write down the reasons why you want to be healthy to keep you on track. Start by adding one new vegetable each week. Walk through the produce section to scout out items you have never tried before. You can go on

Pinterest or Google to discover recipes to use for the new vegetable. My favorite go-to is to peel it, chop it, and roast it in a hot oven (400 degrees) with olive oil, salt, pepper, garlic powder, onion powder, and smoked paprika. Roast until tender.

2. Eat less highly processed foods – avoid/limit store-bought cookies, sugary breakfast cereals, frozen dinners, and snacks. These foods usually have added sugars, unhealthy fats, and a large amount of salt to add flavor and extend shelf life. The healthy parts of the foods – fiber, vitamins, and nutrients have been stripped away.

3. Balance out your plate – Vegetables should be the largest portion on your plate. Look at your plate in fourths. One-half is made up of vegetables. It can be a combination of cooked vegetables and raw vegetables. Raw vegetables such as salads add bulk and fiber to your meal. You will fill up faster with those. One-fourth of your plate should be protein about the size of the palm of your hand. Protein helps you stay fuller longer. The last fourth of the plate can be used for starchy vegetables or whole grains. This is your carbohydrate part. This is the template for a balanced meal.

4. Look for ways to swap healthier choices for less healthy ones – the food industry has listened to

the health experts by producing healthier options. You can use cauliflower rice for regular rice or steam a head of cauliflower until soft. Mash it and prepare it like mashed potatoes. There are kinds of pasta on the label marked *made from lentils or beans.* You can also find vegetables cut into spirals. Use these as a basis for spaghetti sauce. Caution: just get a couple of items to try so you don't end up wasting food. Another tip- if you have any produce that is close to going bad, throw it in a blender. You can use them in a smoothie or in a spaghetti sauce. That is a sneaky way to get more vegetables into your family.

5. Don't eliminate carbohydrates or fats from your meal – Carbohydrates help with satiety. They make you feel good when you eat them. Just be aware of how much you're consuming. Fats add flavor to food. You want to make sure you're eating healthy fats. Fats help to build up healthy cells throughout your body, especially your brain. Fats are also used to produce hormones. So don't strip them from your food.

Macronutrients

Foods are made up of macronutrients and micronutrients. Macronutrients are proteins, fats, and carbohydrates.

Proteins

Proteins are animal or plant–based. As we age, we lose muscle cells. It is important to add protein to each meal to diminish the effects of this loss.

- Animal protein – Beef, poultry, pork, game, seafood, eggs.

- Plant-based protein – Beans, lentils, chickpeas, nuts, soy, tempeh, tofu.

Fats

- Monosaturated – Composed of one carbon. These fats are liquid at room temperature and solidify when chilled. Examples are olive oil and avocado oil.

- Polyunsaturated – Composed of two or more carbon molecules. They are liquid at room temperature. Made up of 2 different types.

  - Omega 3 – this essential fat helps form the cell wall in the body and regulate how they function. A healthy level of omega 3 is needed for hormone production, blood clotting and how the arteries of the body function. Omega 3s can help lower triglycerides in the body.

  - Omega 6 – polyunsaturated fat that helps with skin, hair, and bone health. These fats provide energy.

The key here is the right ratio. There should be more Omega 3 than Omega 6 in the diet. Too much Omega 6 can cause inflammation in the body.

- Saturated – Solid at room temperature. Think butter, coconut oil, or animal fats.

- Trans fats- An industrialized manufactured fat that is used in processed foods. Used in commercial baked goods, snack foods, fried foods, margarine, some oils, and shortening. Using these fats regularly in your foods can raise your cholesterol and increase the risk of heart disease.

Carbohydrates

This is the macronutrient that drives blood sugar. All carbohydrates break down to glucose. Some break down faster than others.

- Simple – also known as sugar. Made of 1 or 2 sugars. Simple carbohydrates breakdown in the body faster and tend to raise your blood sugar fast.

- Complex – also known as starches. Made of multiple sugars. The body digests complex carbohydrates slowly and produces a slow elevation of blood sugars.

- Fiber – there are two categories, and they are complex carbohydrates.

- o Soluble fiber – Breaks down in the small intestine. Provides food for healthy bacteria in the gut. Found in fruits, vegetables, and beans.

- o Insoluble fiber – The body does not digest this fiber. It moves through the intestines and colon. It helps to lower cholesterol. It gives the sensation of fullness when water is consumed. This type of fiber is found in nuts, seeds, and whole grains.

Micronutrients

Micronutrients are the vitamins and minerals contained in the foods we eat. They are in small amounts. Our bodies require small amounts of these nutrients to operate optimally. The absence of these trace minerals can lead to deficiencies and can cause significant illnesses.

The ABCs of A Healthy Meal Plan

- Adequacy – nutrition provides an adequate number of vitamins, minerals, and other nutrients from food. Real food or whole foods are nutritionally dense and generally lower in calories.

- Balance - means that there is a balance of macronutrients and micronutrients in foods consumed. A good meal plan consists of proteins, fats, carbohydrates, vitamins, minerals, and fiber. Eating in this way provides all components needed for healthy living and eliminates cravings because the body is getting everything it needs to operate optimally.

- Calorie Control – Be aware of the number of calories consumed every day. Concentrating on real (whole) food provides fewer calories. An easy method is to eat five servings of vegetables a day. Avoid processed foods that are calorie dense and nutritionally deficient. Processed foods contain unhealthy fats, increased salt, and processed sugars.

- Moderation – No foods are off limits, but we need to limit the amount eaten. Read the label of your favorite snack and find the serving size. Use that as your guide.

- Variety – Variety is the spice of life. Eat a variety of healthy foods, a variety of colors, and different combinations of food to prevent getting bored or burned out on healthy food. Expand your horizon and your palate by trying new foods. Other tools to use are different cooking methods, a new variety of herbs and spices, and sauces.

- Supplements – I recommend taking nutritional supplements because our foods are not as nutritious as they used to be. Vitamins and supplements will be discussed in the medication section.

A Diet You Can Live With

How many times have you started a diet just to fall off the wagon after a few days? Or maybe you were able to stay on it for one month but then fell back into your old eating habits.

Some of us have been successful in losing some weight but then went back to our old eating habits, and before you know it, some of the weight (or all of it) has come back. And they bring friends too. That means more pounds added.

Here are some mindsets, beliefs, or habits that set you up for self-sabotage:

- Being a member of the "Clean Plate Club."
- Taking a nap after eating.
- Must have something sweet after meals.
- Just "a little bit is left, don't throw it away."

Tips to change the above mindsets

- Wait 20 minutes after eating to see if you are really full/satisfied. It takes the brain 20 – 30 minutes to register that there is food in your stomach and that you are full.

- Get only a reasonable portion size – ½ - ¾ cup is the portion size.

- Eat a salad before the meal

- Brush your teeth or use mouthwash after eating.

- Go for a walk after eating.

- For that "spoonful" that's left – throw it away, don't tempt yourself.

- Cravings – usually the body's way of letting you know that there is a deficiency.

- An easy way of preventing cravings – take a multivitamin and vitamin B complex.

- Whole foods vs. processed foods – Whole foods are in their natural state and take longer to digest. Highly processed foods generally have fiber and grains removed to prolong shelf life and make for easier preparation. Most processed foods have added sugar and industrial oils to enhance the flavor.

Healthy Meal Planning

People with diabetes have problems processing starches and sugar. Refined grains such as rice and pasta raise blood sugar fast. Whole grains such as quinoa, brown rice, and whole or old-fashioned oats slowly affect the blood sugar. Fiber recommendations are 25-35 grams /day for women and 35-45 grams/day for men. Fiber promotes a healthy gut and helps to digest food better.

Low Sugar Fruits
- Lemons, limes
- Raspberries
- Strawberries
- Blackberries
- Kiwi
- Grapefruit
- Avocados
- Watermelon

Benefits of Increased Fruit in diet
- Aids digestion
- Boost immune system.
- Decreased risk of colon cancer
- Manages Blood Pressure
- Decreased blood clotting.
- Protects vision, prevents loss.

Eat More of This
Fruits w/edible skin
Raw nuts
Whole grains
Lean protein
Beans and Legumes
Whole grain wrap
Leafy veggies

Eat Less of This
Highly processed foods
Dairy
Sugar sweetened beverages
Trans fats

Benefits of healthy eating
- Increase energy
- Improve sleep

- Better mobility
- Decrease pain
- Increase focus and mental clarity
- Decrease bloating
- Clearer skin
- Better moods

Fun fact: Did you know that taste buds change or regenerate every 2 weeks? If you don't like vegetables, try an experiment. Add one tablespoon of a nonstarchy vegetable to afternoon and evening meal. Then increase it by a tablespoon daily for 2 weeks. See if your taste buds change.

Use fresh or frozen vegetables – use frozen vegetables for affordability and nutrition. Avoid frozen veggies that contain sauces or creams. Choose the ones your family will eat. A few suggestions:

- String beans
- Brussel sprouts
- Broccoli
- Zucchini
- Yellow squash
- Cauliflower - try the riced cauliflower in place of rice.
- Okra

Limit the use of canned foods. They are less nutritious and contain more sodium (salt). There are a few exceptions. They are:

- Beans – black beans, kidney or red beans, white beans, chickpeas

- Tomatoes – processed tomatoes contain lycopene. Lycopene is an antioxidant that provides sun protection, improved heart health, and decrease risk of certain cancers.

Fresh produce
- Salad - bagged salads have a limited shelf life. Check the dates.

- Use romaine lettuce, baby spinach, cucumbers, carrots, and celery for salads.

- Add chopped apple or pear.

Starchy vegetables - limit to ½ cup serving size and eat at mid-day meal.
- Sweet potatoes – fresh ones are cheaper and more nutritious.

- Carrots – Avoid the precut. Whole packaged carrots are cheaper and fresher.

- Hard shell squash- butternut, acorn, spaghetti

- Field peas, lima – frozen are convenient.

- Beets – fresh roasted

Choose whole foods and whole grains. Complex carbs take longer to digest and provides a slow rise of blood sugar. Fiber helps with satiety and sensation of fullness.

- Barley
- oats
- brown rice
- Quinoa

Seasonings – herbs and spices. Try different spices to flavor food to decrease salt use. Increased salt in the diet causes water retention and can raise blood pressure. Seasonings add flavor to the food.

- Smoked paprika in place of smoked meat to flavor vegetable

- Roasted or smoked garlic powder full of flavor

- Use mustard for flavoring meat before cooking.

Mediterranean Diet

The Mediterranean diet is a lifestyle. It is not like other diets that manipulate macros to "force" the body into dropping weight quickly. A true Mediterranean philosophy encompasses not just your eating but other aspects of a healthy life, such as getting regular physical activity and enjoying meals and social time with others.

This diet is full of fiber from legumes and whole grains, high in healthy fats from nuts, seeds, fish, and olive oil, and high in antioxidants from fruits and veggies. These are good for your health. On a

Mediterranean diet, you'll likely to experience less inflammation, better heart health, and more blood sugar control. Frequently, when these measures of health come into alignment, weight loss is a welcome byproduct.

A Mediterranean diet, based on the eating patterns of the populations around the Mediterranean Sea, centers around a menu of whole grains, fruits and vegetables, seafood, plant protein, and minimal dairy. The frequent use of olive oil and moderate red wine consumption are hallmarks of a traditional Mediterranean diet, and it limits sugar and red meat.

Healthy Foods

Whey protein powder is more filling than the soy products and more satisfying than other protein powders. Be sure to read the ingredient labels. Check for fillers and unhealthy products to add bulk.

Yogurt – organic, grass-fed Greek is the best. Grass-fed cows produce omega-3-rich dairy, as opposed to grain or corn - fed produces more omega-6. Greek yogurt is high in protein. Use the plain for the most nutrition. You can add your favorite fruit and toppings for flavor.

Add protein to every meal, including breakfast. Protein will help keep blood sugars stable and keep you fuller longer. Examples of protein are eggs, turkey, chicken, and ground beef. They are cost-effective and can be prepared in many ways. Cheaper cuts of beef contain less fat. These are great for slow-cooker or instant-pot or pressure cooker meals.

Try to avoid barbeque sauce and bottled salad dressing as they contain unhealthy fats and added sugar. There are some healthier versions available, but they can be more expensive. Another option is to make your own. Here is an example of homemade salad dressing. All you need is a jar with a lid. Take ¼ cup olive oil, 2 tablespoons vinegar (any flavor), ½ - 1 teaspoon of soy sauce, and a squirt of mustard. Place in jar and shake. You can add or substitute any of your favorite flavors. Store in the refrigerator. Let it come to room temperature before using.

Avoid the use of canola oil, corn oil, and vegetable oil. These are the unhealthy fats that can lead to clogging of the arteries. Here are some examples of healthy fats to use every day.

- olive oil
- avocado oil
- coconut oil
- Avocado
- Flaxseed
- Tree nuts – walnuts, pecans, pistachios, cashews, almonds

Peanuts are not tree nuts, they are legumes (beans). They are grown in the ground.

Some different ways of increasing vegetables and healthy fats are place roasted vegetable on top of bed of lettuce and sprinkle with ground flaxseed.

Low carbohydrate and Very Low carbohydrate Diets in people with Diabetes

Low-carb diets such as keto have been advocated as an effective method for promoting weight loss for obese individuals and for preventing and treating type 2 diabetes. There are several issues with these plans. In some people, elevated body weight increases the risk of type 2 diabetes, especially if they have been at a normal weight most of their life. Obesity does increase the risk of mortality, such as heart disease, stroke, arthritis, etc. Studies have shown that keto is effective for weight loss in the short term but have shown problems with longevity in living. You can get fast results with keto or low carbohydrate diets, but the issue remains, are you able to stick with that plan long term? Most people revert to their former eating habits once they have reached their goal weight. When that occurs, they end up regaining the weight they lost. Another issue I have observed is muscle loss. When people regain weight, they gain fat and not muscle. My recommendation is losing weight slow and steady. A good rate is 1- 2 pounds per week.

The onset and progression of obesity and type 2 diabetes can be delayed with:

- Exercise
- Diet
- Weight loss of 5-10% of body weight

Type 2 diabetes is a lifestyle-mediated chronic disease. The emphasis is on dietary modification and a determined effective eating plan. That is translated to a diet or plan that you can stick with.

Meal planning should be tailored to your eating patterns, preference, and metabolic goals. I do not advocate using popular or trendy diet plans unless you can stick with them for the long term. If it is a new lifestyle for you, go for it. But as a rule of thumb, quick weight loss can lead to quick weight regain.

Label Reading

Reading labels will help you to determine if a food is healthy for you or not.

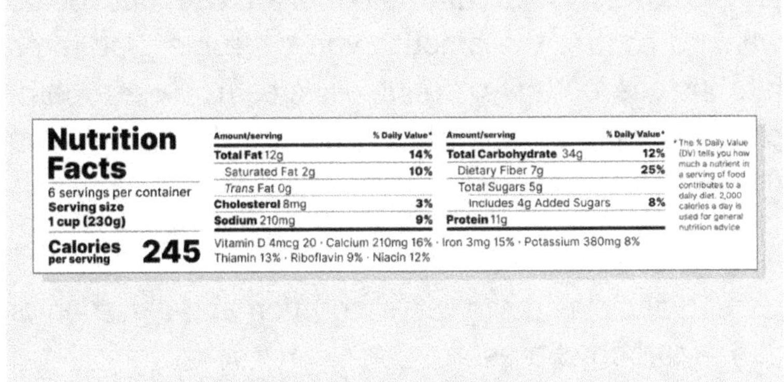

Nutrition Facts	Amount/serving	% Daily Value*	Amount/serving	% Daily Value*	
	Total Fat 12g	**14%**	**Total Carbohydrate** 34g	**12%**	*The % Daily Value (DV) tells you how much a nutrient in a serving of food contributes to a daily diet. 2,000 calories a day is used for general nutrition advice
	Saturated Fat 2g	**10%**	Dietary Fiber 7g	**25%**	
6 servings per container	Trans Fat 0g		Total Sugars 5g		
Serving size	**Cholesterol** 8mg	**3%**	Includes 4g Added Sugars	**8%**	
1 cup (230g)	**Sodium** 210mg	**9%**	**Protein** 11g		
Calories per serving **245**	Vitamin D 4mcg 20 · Calcium 210mg 16% · Iron 3mg 15% · Potassium 380mg 8% Thiamin 13% · Riboflavin 9% · Niacin 12%				

We will use the above illustration for an example. This is a nutrition label. The important areas are how many servings per container, serving size, total fat, sodium which is the salt content, and total carbohydrates. The amounts listed is per serving, not for the whole container.

I will cover carbohydrates first because that is what drives blood sugars. The total carbohydrates are broken down into categories – dietary fiber, total sugars which includes added sugars. Here's a tip, the higher the fiber content, the better. The fiber in foods passes through the body to aid in digestion or in fullness. Fiber provides food or nutrients for the gut. That helps to improve gut health.

Fat on the nutrition label is broken down into saturated fats and trans fats. You want to avoid trans fats as much as possible. Trans fats are those unhealthy fats that can clog up your arteries. Saturated fats are the ones that are solid at room temperature. Not all saturated fats are bad, but you do want to control the amount you consume. Saturated fats include butter, coconut oil, cream, cheese, lard, palm oil, and cocoa butter. The benefits of fat in a product are:

- Fat adds flavor
- Fat slows down the absorption and digestion of carbohydrates.
- Fat gives the body energy

- Fat helps with absorption of important vitamins – A, D, E, K
- Fat helps with the production of hormones in the body

The amount of protein in a product is helpful to prolonging fullness and protein is essential in building up the cells of the body, especially muscles. Adding protein to your meals is a safeguard against mindless snacking and eating between meals. The protein, fiber, and fat will help keep you fuller longer.

You want to control the amount of salt or sodium in your diet and foods. On the nutrition label you want 200 mg or less. Too much salt in a product can lead to fluid retention and swelling. We do need some salt in our diet to balance our electrolytes but not too much.

The real information is on the ingredient label or like I say, the devil is in the details. The ingredient list is the small print under the nutrition label or on the side of the container. By law ingredients are listed by its common name and in descending order by weight. There are four classes of sweeteners.

- Sugars
  - Brown sugar
  - Corn syrup, includes high fructose
  - Molasses
  - Honey
  - Sucrose – table sugar

- o Fructose
- o Maltose

- Sugar alcohols – Products that contain these are labeled as "sugar free"
  - o Erythritol
  - o Mannitol
  - o Sorbitol
  - o Xylitol

- Artificial sweeteners
  - o Sucralose - Splenda
  - o Saccharin – Sweet and Low
  - o Aspartame - Equal
  - o Acesulfame – Sweet One

- Natural low calorie sweeteners
  - o Stevia
  - o Monk fruit

High fructose corn syrup is the industrial sweetener made from corn. It is cheap and it does sweeten. That is the sweeteners most used in sodas, juices, candy, etc. The health problem high fructose corn syrup presents are it goes to the liver. As opposed to sugar/glucose that is absorbed by the muscles and other cells. Increased use of high fructose corn syrup has led to many cases of nonalcoholic fatty liver disease. This condition left unchecked and untreated can progress to cirrhosis of the liver and then to liver cancer. So that is why there has been a big push to eliminate the use of high fructose corn syrup and replace it with cane sugar. But our aim is to limit all sugars as much as possible. You still need to inspect your ingredient labels. Always check the ingredient label. The big print on the front of the product can be misleading. No sugar added can mean there's artificial sweeteners in it, such as sucralose or aspartame. Look for sugar alcohol ingredients in products labeled sugar free. Even with the low calorie sweeteners check the ingredient label. Manufacturers have mixed in other sugars in with the low-calorie sweeteners. For example, Stevia in the Raw contains dextrose and stevia leaf extract, Truvia contains erythritol, stevia leaf extract, and other natural flavors. Beware of eating a large amount of "sugar free" products. The sugar alcohols are the same components used in laxatives.

Another ingredient to be on the lookout for is fats.

- Beef fat
- Butter
- Coconut
- Coconut oil
- Cream
- Full cream mild powder
- Ghee
- Hydrogenated oils
- Lard
- Mayonnaise
- Mono-di-or triglycerides

- Palm oil
- Shortening
- Suet
- Tallow
- Vegetable oil

Hydrogenated oils, partially hydrogenated oils, vegetable oils are the ones that contribute to raising LDL levels. The problem with these fats, the body cannot fully digest them. I recommend natural products over manmade every time. Butter and ghee are all natural products with little processing. Always buy the best products you can afford. Organic, grass-fed is the best but if it is out of your price range, go with the next best product. That would be butter. When choosing or comparing a product, the rule of thumb is the shorter the ingredient list the better. The longer list generally has longer names that are difficult to pronounce. If you can't pronounce it, stay away from it. This rule applies to convenience foods, too.

Shopping Tips and Meal Prep
The best way to stay on track with your meal preparation is to plan out your menu for the week before you go shopping. If you are cooking for your family, get them involved in the menu planning stage. That will keep down the refusal of eating the meals. If you have diabetes, the risk of your family developing diabetes is high. So, it is in their best interest to eat the same meals as you eat.

Another tip is to check your cabinets, pantry, refrigerator, and freezer to see what you have on hand. Doing a pre-shopping inventory will avoid buying duplicates. That way you will not have products on the shelf for years. You want to rotate your stock to keep things fresh. Make your list to take while shopping. You can write the list out and take a picture with your phone so you will always have the list. To stay within your budget, check the grocery ads to see what is on sale. You can adjust your menu to fit what is on sale. Make sure you eat before going to the store. You will sabotage your budget if you go to shopping without eating. Everything will look good and tempting while you're shopping.

While shopping stick to the perimeter/outside of the store. That is where the produce section, meat and seafood, dairy and fresh products are kept.

Points to remember

- Buy the best products that you can afford. Don't spend extra money if you can't afford it.

- Organic vegetables and fruits are more affordable if bought frozen

- Fresh produce - no need to buy organic if product must be peeled

- Buy produce in season

- Farmers markets are usually more affordable, grown locally

- Organic or whole grain products have a shorter shelf life, so plan to use it or freeze to preserve it

- If you buy too much at one time - take time to package and freeze it for later use.

- Remember food is fuel for your body. Provide the best you can for your family.

Aisle shopping - Allowable

* Seasonings

- Garlic powder, roasted, granulated
- Onion powder
- Italian seasoning or Herbes de' Provence
- Single herb seasoning cumin, chili powder, red pepper, turmeric
- Salad dressings - vinaigrettes, olive oil and vinegar, balsamic - avoid products with soybean and canola oil
- Nuts - raw almonds, walnuts, pistachios, cashews, pecans
- Stock or broth - chicken, beef, veggie. Low sodium
- Bone broth - good for warm snack or add veggies for soup
- Beans - dried or canned (labeled BPA). Plain beans, not seasoned

- Nut butter - natural - peanut, almond, cashew, etc.
- Salmon - canned or fresh, wild caught
- Tuna - canned or fresh
- Sardines or fish steaks, canned

Produce Department
- Chopped veggies
- Bagged fresh veggies
- Whole fruits and veggies
- Fresh herbs
- Salad dressings - Yogurt based - without soybean or canola oil
- Avocado - healthy fat
- Seasonal veggies are generally cheaper

Meat Department
- Fresh prepped meals
- Seasoned meats
- Bacon - nitrate-free
- Fresh sausage - bratwurst, Italian
- Fresh lean beef, pork, lamb, veal
- Chicken, turkey.
- Fish and seafood- wild caught is best

Frozen foods
- Veggies without sauce
- Fruit without added sugar or juices
- Cold water fish - cod, halibut, grouper
- Shrimp - wild caught. Feeds on vegetation in water

Dairy

- Yogurt, plain
- Kefir, plain
- Cheese - full fat
- Cream Cheese
- Fresh tortillas
- Eggs

Deli Department

- Hummus
- Guacamole
- Premade salads - green - the salad dressings in the pack are not the healthiest
- Organic, nitrate, and antibiotic free deli meats
- Salsa

Products to Avoid

- Avoid use of bouillon cubes and Better than bouillon - MSG content
- Canned soups - sodium and different additives
- Canned seasoned beans and vegetables - increased salt and other additive
- Low-fat products - usually has added sugar to add flavor
- Low sugar, no sugar added products
- Luncheon meats - nitrites and other additives that cause inflammation.
- Season mixtures - Salt is usually the first ingredient

- Farm- raised seafood - feed is usually GMO (genetically modified) grain
- Low -fat Peanut butter - additives and added sugar.
- Nonmeat products - look at ingredients, many contain fillers and non-nutritive additives.
- Sausages and hot dogs - low protein and increase additives, unless pure beef for hot dogs and pure pork, chicken, or beef for sausage
- Tofu - GMO products
- Cheese in a can
- Low-fat/no fat cheeses - little nutritional value and increased additives
- Juices - too much sugar
- Egg beaters
- Nonfat, low-fat salad dressings -increased additives to add flavor
- Flavored yogurts - fruit added, nonfat. Too much sugar and other additives.
- Canola oil, vegetable oil, corn oil - GMO products, causes inflammation

Now to make your meals
Breakfast
- Protein - eggs, leftover meats such as baked poultry, beef, or pork. Ground turkey is a go-to. Word of caution – most people substitute turkey products for pork. Read the labels. Turkey

products contain preservatives and large amounts of sodium. An alternative can be grass-fed, organic products. They may cost more, but they are a healthier product. Look for sales.

- Complex carbs – whole grain toast, oatmeal, beans, quinoa, sweet potatoes, barley
- Healthy fats –avocados, pecans, walnuts, pistachios, almonds, coconut, ground flaxseed. Limit use to 2 tablespoons

Lunch - make this your heavier meal.

Eating your heavier meal midday gives you plenty of time to burn off the calories and lower blood sugar.

- Protein -serving size of the palm of a hand.
- Starchy carb - limit to ½ cup
- Non-starchy veggie, salad- unlimited amounts
- Healthy fat- 2 tablespoon

Dinner – try to eat 3 hours before bed.

Eating in this manner gives your body time to fully digest the food.

- Protein - serving size of the palm of a hand.
- Non starchy veggies, add a salad for bulk and fullness.
- Avoid starchy carbs for the evening meal.
- Healthy fat – 2 tablespoons

Hydration – Your Choice of Beverage

Hydration is important, especially as you get older. It's even more important if you have diabetes. The goal is for you to match your drink choices, your lifestyle, your taste preferences, and your plan.

If your goal is to lose weight, increase your water intake. The ideal is ½ your body weight in fluid ounces per day. For example, if you weigh 180 pounds, water would be 90 ounces daily. If you don't drink much water, slowly increase the amount you drink. After a couple of weeks, look at how you feel. Increased water intake promotes increased waste removal. The water will flush out the toxins in your body.

If you're a committed soda drinker, try substituting with no–calorie sparkling water. Mix it with a splash of your favorite juice to flavor it. We want to help you succeed.

Other acceptable beverages are tea and coffee. One endocrinologist recommended black currant tea. It helps to lower and stabilize blood sugar. Another bonus is it helps to promote sleep. Recommendation for alcohol. For women, no more than one drink a day. Men are limited to two drinks a day. The drink serving sizes are beer 12 ounces, wine 5 ounces, and liquor 1.5 ounces.

Exercise – The Original Fountain of Youth

Exercise is the 3rd pillar of healthy living. This is especially important as we age. A friend of mine posted this. "Fad diets can change your weight; working out can change your body."

Functional fitness is doing movements using multiple muscle groups to help with daily activities. Walking is the easiest and cheapest form of functional fitness. Walking for functional fitness increases your heart rate and improves your oxygen use. It also helps to improve circulation and muscle strength.

An Example of Functional Fitness and Longevity

I had a clinic in a rural area in Alabama. There was a 70-year-old lady who would walk 2 miles every day. One day I decided to walk with her. I could not keep up with her. She walked so fast that I had difficulty keeping up with her. Afterward, she told me that she started walking after she was diagnosed with cancer. Her walking program started while undergoing treatment for colon cancer. She walked daily, even though she was going through treatment, even when she didn't feel well. Her walking program improved her quality of life and increased her lifespan. The functional fitness benefit she derived from walking is health maintenance and well-being. Walking increases your lifespan. You will naturally improve your life expectancy by just walking. Your quality of life can improve according to the goals you have set.

Functional Fitness and Weight Management

Another benefit is walking manages your weight. Functional fitness by walking increases calorie burn and improves aerobic capacity. The benefit you derive from walking depends on how far you walk, how often you walk, and how fast you walk. A good pace needs to be fast enough so that you can talk but are not able to sing. Consistency is the key to a successful walking program.

When you exercise and use your muscles, you are using energy. Your body must use something for energy. When you walk on an empty stomach, your body may use stored fat as fuel or energy. Walking builds up muscle cells, which is good for the body because muscle cells are active even at rest. Muscle cells help to burn fat. An effective walking program can shave inches off your body. It will build up muscle cells in your body.

Functional fitness can prevent dementia

Functional fitness improves aerobic capacity. That means that your body uses oxygen better. Increased oxygen improves circulation to the brain, which in turn can reduce the risk of dementia. Dementia is caused by plaque build-up in the brain. Walking increases your blood circulation. Increased circulation increases the flow of oxygen. When you increase blood circulation to your brain, the plaques cannot settle. So, increased blood flow leads to increased oxygen and a decrease in plaque formation, therefore a little risk of developing dementia.

Functional fitness and increased mobility

Functional fitness improves joint health. Walking is an activity that is easy on the joints. Walking increases the lubrication of the joints. Functional fitness and increased mobility involve squatting down to pick up objects or reach to get items off a shelf.

Walking is better for the joints than jogging or running. Walking puts less pressure and exertion on the joints.

Functional fitness includes safety in movement. Walking strengthens your bones and reduces your risk of osteoporosis. Bones can become weaker as you age, especially in post-menopausal women or had a hysterectomy. Women lose the protection of estrogen when they age. There's an increased risk of osteopenia, and osteoporosis, a weakening of the bones. But when you walk, you're putting stress on your legs, and we call it weight-bearing exercises. And that causes those limbs to strengthen. That strengthening improves your functional fitness.

Functional Fitness and Restorative Sleep

Functional fitness improves restorative sleep. Restorative sleep is when you feel rested and refreshed after sleeping at night. Walking improves your sleep by allowing pent-up emotions and frustrations to be released. Walking helps to restore your body and your mind.

Functional Fitness and Muscle Tone

Walking tones, your legs, your butt, and your stomach. Functional fitness involves building muscle tone and strength. The tone helps to improve your posture when you're walking. Using those lower extremity muscles is a game changer in functional fitness.

Functional Fitness and Women over 50

Building up functional fitness in women over 50 is essential for good health. Diabetes, pre-diabetes, or any chronic health problem is more prominent in the over-50 age group. So, it is important to focus on building up your functional fitness.

The danger of not exercising is the increased risk of adverse health outcomes, including weight gain and obesity, heart disease, type 2 diabetes, metabolic syndrome, and increased risk of some cancers. Bodies are made to move. The more sedentary you are, the more danger of disease and premature aging.

2-weeks of inactivity can cause significant health problems, loss of muscle mass, and metabolic changes can occur. That is why they get you up and moving while in the hospital. Studies have shown it is important to focus on a greater frequency of movement throughout the entire day. Aim for 3-6 minutes of movement every hour. Consider this an exercise snack.

How to identify a sedentary lifestyle
8 signs you're not physically active enough.

1. You fall short of global health recommendations – 150 – 300 minutes moderate–intensity aerobic activity per week or 75-150 of vigorous–intensity aerobic activity per week, plus two days of strength training. If you are not meeting either of these, you are not moving enough.

2. You spend more than half your waking hours not moving – hours of sleep – 24 hours. If you spend more than 50% of your time sitting, reclining, and not moving. Find ways to change this.

3. A fatigued feeling all the time – fatigue comes from stress, poor diet, and hormone imbalances. Being more sedentary leads to being deconditioned (heart, lungs, muscles). People who did 20 minutes of low or medium-intensity exercise 3x/week for 6-weeks experienced a 20% energy boost.

4. Changes in weight and metabolism – weight fluctuation. Too many sedentary practices and eating the same amount leads to increased fat production. A sedentary

lifestyle affects metabolism. The blood flow is slowed down and results in slower metabolism. Long-term sedentary lifestyle can lead to type 2 diabetes, heart attack, stroke, and other chronic diseases.

5. You often feel winded or short of breath – Your breathing becomes shallow. This leads to less oxygen being delivered throughout the body and returning to the heart. Over time you can develop a deconditioned heart. Minimal movement can make you feel winded faster, and you may experience palpitations which indicates heart deterioration and function.

6. You have trouble sleeping – The recommended amount is 7-9 hours per night. Not getting enough sleep can lead to metabolism issues, a weakened immune system, and increased risk of early death. The more inactive you are, the more your sleep will suffer. Sedentary 11 hours or more leads to reduced sleep quality and sleep quantity.

7. You notice that your mental health has diminished. The more sedentary you are leads to decreased psychological well-being and quality of life. It also leads to more depression. Exercise is associated with the release of serotonin (feel good hormones).

The more serotonin you have will cause you to crave exercise and commit to exercise plans. Serotonin is that hormone that bring a lightened mood and increased joy. Exercise can reverse depression.

8. Impaired memory – the brain needs exercise. Hours spent sitting leads to less thickness of the medial temporal lobe, where memory is housed. Add aerobic activity, like walking. This helps with delay of age-related cognitive issues like dementia. Small changes lead to big results.

The more stagnant you are, the greater risk of mortality and heart disease. Increased TV watching leads to increased heart disease risk. The older you are, the longer it takes to recover from a sedentary state. But 8-10 weeks of consistent workouts can recondition the heart. Here are some examples to recondition your heart and improve your health.

- Start by walking for 10 minutes every other day – start and be consistent.

- The goal is to work up to 30 minutes of moderate-intensity exercise 5 days/week. The ultimate goal is 150 minutes per week.

- Light–intensity movement for 1-5 minutes every hour can make a significant impact.

- For additional health benefits, add weightlifting exercises 2-3 times a week. Start using light weights to exercises. Weights will rebuild muscle cells in the body. Muscle development can halt sarcopenia, which is age -related progressive loss of muscle mass and strength.

There are many exercises for seniors and women over 50 on YouTube. That way you can exercise in the comfort and convenience of your home. If you have problems with mobility, there are even chair exercises available.

Becoming aware of underactive tendencies and choosing to be active can help put your mind and mood in a better position. Mindfulness is crucial. Mindfulness can strengthen your ability to combat stress and anxiety. The habit of moving is extremely beneficial to optimizing the relationship between fitness and mental health. Being mindful of being active can lift the mood and lessen stress. The effects are amplified when both things are practiced together.

Effective Sleep is fundamental

Sleep is the 4th pillar of healthy living. I intend to help you and give information you can use to make sure that you age gracefully. With aging, you are more prone to health problems. You want to lower the risk of complications from chronic disease. Sleep is a vital aspect of health living.

Stages of Sleep

- Stage One –This is the transition between wakefulness and sleep. This stage lasts about five to 10 minutes.

- Stage two – Stage of quiet sleep. During this stage, your temperature drops. The breathing and heart rate decrease and become more regular. Your brain produces sleep spindles at this stage. Sleep spindles are like memory cells. This stage lasts for about 20 minutes.

- Stage three - The stages between light sleep and very deep sleep. At this stage, blood pressure drops, and your breathing rate slows even more. Your sleep deepens to the restful sleep stage. Body restoration and repair occur during this stage.

- Stage four – Active sleep stage or REM stage. REM stands for rapid eye movement. Even though your brain is more active, this is another stage of deep, restorative sleep. Hormone production and muscle repair occurs during this stage. Melatonin is produced during this stage. It is a natural hormone the body produces to induce sleep. Melatonin needs a dark environment for production. Memories are sorted and filed during this stage.

The ideal amount of sleep is 7-9 hours of sleep. Less than 6 hours have been shown to produce problems with weight, blood sugar control, and blood pressure regulation.

Sleep Disruption

Several issues can disrupt your sleep. One issue is if you have a spouse or partner you sleep with. If your partner is a restless sleeper or a snorer, that can disrupt your sleep.

Another thing to consider as being older than 50 is hormonal changes, especially in women. Loss of estrogen can lead to an increase in cortisol production. Cortisol release can disrupt sleep. One of the changes that happens with aging, there's less time in the deep sleep stage.

Blood sugars and blood pressure tend to be out of control with sleep disturbances. Sleep apnea or obstructive sleep apnea can cause sleep disruption or sleep disturbances. This obstruction can prevent you from going into a deep sleep cycle because the body has built-in protective mechanisms. So, if you find that you are tired when you wake up and feel like you haven't slept at all, you may need to talk to your provider about it because you may need to have a sleep study done. Something proactive you can do is to have a nighttime routine.

We call it sleep hygiene. This is a routine. So, you can have a routine that allows your body to start slowing down and getting ready for sleep

The routine consists of:

- Turn off your electronics at least one to two hours before bedtime. The blue light that emits from cell phones, computer, and TV causes the brain to continue being active. Refrain from checking your email, social media, and text messages during this time.

- Some things that can help promote sleep are reading a book that is relaxing or listening to soothing music to calm you before going to sleep.

- Another thing is don't eat for three hours before bed. Eating too close before going to bed can interfere with sleep. Your body is awake during the night to digest the food that you have eaten. You cannot go into a deep sleep because it will slow down the digestive process. The digestion is still working. Some people like warm milk or tea before bed. These drinks may not disturb your sleep. In fact, it may promote sleepiness. Be mindful of consuming other liquids before going to bed. Liquids before bed may cause you to have to use the bathroom during the night.

- Avoid strenuous exercise or increased activity too close to bedtime, except sexual intercourse. Activity is not conducive to a good night's sleep. What may be helpful is meditation or yoga, which is relaxing to promote sleep.

- A busy brain can interfere with sleep. A busy brain is too many things on your mind. Write down your thoughts or concerns. We call it a brain dump. That is a way of letting go of what's on your mind. Another practice is making a gratitude journal. Write down things that you're grateful for.

Sleep impairment leads to insulin resistance which is a precursor to prediabetes and type two diabetes. So do all you can to improve your quality of sleep so health problems can be avoided. Your sleep is conducive to healthy aging.

Stress Management

Stress management is the 5th pillar. As long as we live, we will have some type of stress. The key is how we respond and manage it. There are three types of stress.

1. Acute Stress - Sudden onset, short-lived. Fight or flight response. It is a protective type of response. Examples- a sudden stop in traffic to prevent impact, a child going to a dangerous

object or situation. Immediate response is to cortisol release, heart racing, hard breathing, and eyes open wide.

2. Recurrent acute stress – Series of stressful situations occurring. It's more of a controlled response.

3. Chronic stress – Think of this as a slow burn. You get the feeling of overwhelm and pressure. Relationships, work-related issues, environmental concerns, and PTSD are examples of chronic stress. Unaddressed or unopposed chronic stress promotes chronic health problems. Chronic stress can lead to anxiety, insomnia, problems with blood pressure control, and a weakened immune system. Your blood sugar reacts to stress in your body and environment.

Foods that make stress worse

- Highly processed foods
- Fast food
- Commercial baked goods – cakes, cookies because they contain polyunsaturated fatty acids. These are the unhealthy or industrialized fats.

Foods that improve stress

- Oily fish – salmon, tuna, anchovies, sardines are examples
- Shellfish – shrimp, scallops, crab, oysters, lobster
- Vitamin C – fruits and vegetables
- Multicolored vegetables
- Beans and legumes

The best way to eat to relieve stress

- Take the time to eat in a relaxed atmosphere.
- Be mindful of what you eat.
- Pay attention to your body.
- Distinguish and recognize the difference between physical and emotional hunger – become more aware of your body
- Avoid multi-tasking – avoid electronic distractions while eating.
- Slow down – take time to savor food, chew slowly.

Another stress reliever is journaling. Writing about an unpleasant topic diffuses it and removes the power it has over you. It can help decrease adverse health reactions.

Chapter 7: Build Your Healthcare Team

No man (woman) is an island. In a multitude of counselors (or providers), there is much wisdom. A well-rounded healthcare team has you, the client, at the center. Your primary care provider, endocrinologist, ophthalmologist, podiatrist, dentist, pharmacist, nephrologist, dietician, and diabetes educator are essential team members.

Primary Care provider (PCP)– May be a medical doctor, nurse practitioner, or physician assistant. Choose a PCP that you can talk to, one that will listen to what you have to say and adjust the care plan to fit your needs. A good PCP will recommend and inform you of a particular treatment and assure you that it's in your best interest. A caring PCP will consider your insurance coverage and ability to afford the care. Not all PCPs are created equal. Not all providers are up to date on diabetes care and treatment. So, consider finding one that has an interest in caring for you.

Endocrinologist –A medical doctor that specializes diagnosing and treating diabetes, thyroid conditions, metabolic conditions, and other hormone producing organs. Referrals to endocrinologists is warranted if the PCP is not successful in controlling the diabetes.

Ophthalmologist – An ophthalmologist is a physician that specializes in the eye. It is essential for you to have regular eye exams – especially dilated exams. The dilation allows the doctor to look at the compartment behind the eye to ensure there's no bleeding or plaques. I recommend an ophthalmologist exam in addition to an optician. The optician is good for measuring and prescribing glasses. An ophthalmologist does a more detailed eye and retinal exam.

Diabetic retinopathy is caused by bleeding behind the eye. This is one of the common complications of uncontrolled diabetes. The danger is you do not notice any changes in your vision in the early stages. Left untreated, permanent eye damage and blindness can occur. Retinopathy can be treated by drops and injections. The number one way to control retinopathy is controlling your blood sugar.

Other common eye problems that can occur are glaucoma and cataracts. Glaucoma is increased pressure in the eye that can press on the optic nerve. Untreated pressure for a prolonged time can lead to blindness. Treatment after early detection of glaucoma is with eye drops and/or laser surgery. Regular eye exams are the most important to ensure the pressures remain at acceptable levels.

Cataracts are another complication and are caused by inflammation. This inflammation is a result persistent elevated blood sugar. Cataracts are a cloudiness of the lens in the eye. Age-related cataracts are the most common type but uncontrolled diabetes at a younger age can lead to cataracts. Ophthalmology visits are usually every six months unless there is a problem that requires close follow-up.

Podiatrist- A doctor that specializes in treatment of variety of foot and ankle problems. You should have a good podiatrist on your team. You only get one pair of feet and protecting them should be your priority. Podiatry visits are generally every 8 -12 weeks for inspection, sensation and nerve assessment along with nail and foot care. You should never clip your own toenails because you can nick your skin or cut nails too short and cause injury. Skin wounds and injuries in people with diabetes can lead to infection. The danger of foot problems comes from poor circulation.

Your feet are the farthest away from your heart, and blood flow may be impaired. Another problem that occurs is nerve damage, called neuropathy. Neuropathy is a consequence of longstanding diabetes. You must inform your PCP and podiatrist of any numbness, tingling, or pain in your feet. You must avoid soaking your feet in hot water unless you check the temperature with a thermometer or inner arm. Don't trust using your feet as a gauge because of impaired sensation. If you don't have insurance and cannot afford to see a podiatrist, there are some tasks that you can do yourself, but please follow the recommendations given.

Dentist – Dental care is important because your mouth harbors many bacteria. Poor dental and poor gum health can contribute to high blood sugars. Missing and decayed teeth prevent you from chewing your food completely and getting all its nutrients. Plaque builds up on the teeth and leads to gum disease and can cause chronic infection of the gums. Regular dental checkups can decrease the risk of these problems. Periodic full dental cleaning keeps the plaque cleared. These checkups provide an opportunity for a full mouth exam. Mouth cancer starts as an irregularity on or under the tongue or the palate. These first lesions are usually not painful. Just like everything else, early detection is important.

Nephrologist – This is a medical doctor that specializes in kidney health and treatment. You may need a referral to a nephrologist if your kidney function is declining. The nephrologist will be able to prescribe medications and/or treatment to preserve your kidney function. The goal is to avoid dialysis.

Pharmacist – You should have a dedicated pharmacy and pharmacist. Your pharmacist has all your medications and any documented allergies on record. This is vital because they will be able to alert any provider of any potential drug interactions or duplicates. A dedicated pharmacist will give you the best price and provide the best benefits for you. They will also alert you when phoned in prescriptions are not covered by insurance. For example, I got a refill on my blood pressure medicine, and they gave me 30 days. They let me know there was not a copay for 30-day refills but there was a charge for 90-day refills. It will benefit you to establish a rapport with your pharmacy staff. Now most pharmacies provide vaccinations so that is another area where your medications are documented.

Dietician – A food and nutrition expert whose focus is to keep the client healthy. They can be certified as diabetes educator. The dietician will evaluate your nutritional needs, make meal plan recommendations, and provide counseling to improve your health.

Diabetes Educator – The formal name is diabetes care and education specialist. This individual can be a nurse, doctor, pharmacist, or nutritionist. They are a vital part of your healthcare team. They provide evidence – based self-management education and programs. They teach skills and strategies needed to manage and control diabetes. The teaching they provide depends on their training and occupation. A nutritionist/dietician can provide detailed information on foods and meal planning. A diabetes educator can be that go - to person to provide education, support, and coaching to help you set your goals and determine your action steps.

Chapter 8: Medication Management

Medications usually used by people with diabetes are blood pressure, cholesterol, and diabetes medications. Blood pressure medications are used to control blood pressure and increase blood circulation to the kidneys.

There are several classes of cholesterol medications. The goal of therapy is to lower the LDL (bad). People with diabetes and people over 50 are at higher risk of plaque accumulation. That plaque accumulation can lead to coronary artery disease. The proactive approach is to take a statin to lower LDL and stabilize your vessels. There are cases where people cannot tolerate statins so alternative therapy is recommended. Lifestyle behavior change such as diet and exercise changes are vital to contribute to decreasing problems. The goal of therapy is to prevent acute coronary episode, such as heart attack or stroke. That is why your providers are sticklers about all of your medications.

Diabetes medications

- **Metformin** – This medicine makes the body more sensitive to its natural insulin. Generally, it's the first-line choice. It can cause nausea and diarrhea when you first start it. That's why I recommend taking it before your largest meal, starting at the lowest dose. Metformin does not cause your blood sugar to drop. Vitamin B12 is recommended, but I recommend vitamin B complex. The B complex ensures that you will have a balance of all the B vitamins. There are natural alternatives to Metformin called Berberine. Cost $

- **Sulfonylureas Glipizide/Glyburide** – These medications work on the pancreas, stimulating it to produce more insulin. These medications can cause blood sugars to drop. Glyburide is not recommended if there is chronic kidney disease. These are not favored medications because prolong use can cause pancreas to become exhausted. Just like wringing water out of a dishrag. There comes a time when no water is left. The same with the pancreas, there may come a time when there's no insulin produced. Cost $

- **TZD (Actos, Avandia)** – This medication improves insulin sensitivity in the body by decreasing glucose release from the liver. It also causes the fat and muscle cells to increase the use of blood sugar. People with congestive heart failure, and kidney problems cannot use this medication because it causes fluid retention. Cost $

- **DPP-4 Inhibitors (Januvia, Janumet, Onglyza)** – This is one of the first "smart" drugs. It will stimulate the release of insulin after eating. It will not stimulate insulin if it is not needed. The insulin released works directly on glucose. It also inhibits the release of stored glucose in the liver. Cost $$$

- **GLP agonist (Injectables Victoza, Byetta, Ozempic, Saxenda, Adlyxin)** – Controls blood sugar by increasing insulin production after eating. It also slows stomach emptying. Decreased appetite occurs, which leads to weight loss. This may cause nausea, vomiting, and diarrhea. People that have heart disease benefit from taking this medication. This medication is preferred for second line after Metformin if A1C is elevated. Cost $$$

- **SGLT I (Injectables Jardiance, Invokana, Farxiga, Trulicity; pill Rybelsus)** – These medications lower blood sugar by directing glucose to kidneys to be excreted. This medicine does not stimulate insulin production. These medications protect the kidneys by improving kidney metabolism. They also promote weight loss. Many are using this medication for weight loss and not for diabetes. Cost $$$

- **Insulin – Injections**. There are many different types of insulin on the market. The most commonly used insulins are long acting or basal and short acting or bolus. The purpose of the insulin is to mimic the body's natural insulin. The basal insulin is released slowly throughout the day. They are generally used once a day. The bolus insulin is used before meals and for correcting high blood sugars. Insulin is used by people with type 2 diabetes if other medications have not been effective in controlling blood sugars. Insulin can be used in combination with other medications to control diabetes. The cost of insulin varies according to type of insulin and third-party payor. Cost ranges $ - $$$

Medications can help control diabetes and improve quality of life. Vitamins and supplements are beneficial in controlling blood sugars and preventing problems with deficiencies. Some of the supplements and recommendations are explained. This is just a sampling of products on the market.

- Always start with a good multivitamin. It will provide the foundation needed for health and prevent shortages in different areas.

- Vitamin D3 – It is essential for heart and bone health.

- Vitamin B complex – best contain methylated B12

- Alpha lipoic acid – this is an antioxidant that treats oxidative stress. Oxidative stress is caused by buildup of toxic substances in the body. The body is unable to eliminate all these substances, thereby causing an imbalance. These harmful substances can cause kidney or nerve damage, leading to chronic kidney disease or neuropathy. Alpha lipoic acid helps to eliminate some of these harmful substances.

- Benfotiamine – this is a form of vitamin B1. Essential for nerve health. May help decrease pain of neuropathy

- Omega 3 fish oil – provides healthy fat needed for hormone and cell production

- Co enzyme Q10 – this is an antioxidant that get depleted with use of statins and /or Metformin

- Magnesium glycinate– helps to control blood pressure and blood sugar. It also promotes rest and helps with sleep. Magnesium can be depleted with use of diuretics (water pills) and Metformin.

- Rhodiola – herbal medicine called adaptogen. It helps to relieve stress and anxiety. It can boost your energy and help with physical performance. Do not take if taking prescription antidepressants or other mental health medications.

- Ashwagandha – this is an herbal medicine called adaptogens. It helps to relieve stress and anxiety. Ashwagandha provides more relaxation. It is not recommended if you are taking antidepressants or other mental health medications.

I recommend buying good quality supplements. I caution to avoid the bargain ones. The brands I recommend are:

- Pure Encapsulations – most products are in capsule form for easy digestion and absorption.

- Thorne – they make good quality products but are pricier.

- Life Extension – they too make good products and less pricey.

The thing about supplements is they are to supplement a healthy diet. Some should only be used for a short period of time. Don't try to substitute your prescription medicine with supplements on your own. Always discuss ANY and ALL medications, prescription, or supplement with your provider. Your provider should know what medications you are taking. There are providers that are unaware of the benefits of supplements. The argument most providers have about supplements are lack of controlled studies and trials. Another argument is supplements are not regulated by the government. That is why I recommend certain products. I stand by their products. They provide studies to back their claims.

81

Chapter 9: Prevent Diabetes-Related Complications

Smoking Cessation - One of the first things or habits to quit is smoking. Tobacco use is linked to many health problems and risks that quitting is in your best interest. Plus, it is so expensive. If you have problems quitting, some programs and assistance are available.

Smoking increases the risk of cancer. Throat, lung, breast, and bladder, to name a few. Another problem with smoking is the expense. If you have problems getting your medications, buying healthy food, or paying for provider visits, look at how much you spend on smoking. Lastly, smoking affects your circulation and blood vessels. That is why smokers complain of cold extremities and decreased sensation.

Head to Toe Self-care
Mouth care – Regular brushing your teeth, flossing, and using mouthwash will help keep your mouth

clean and decrease germs and bacteria. Your teeth need special care because that is how you chew your food adequately to get all the nutrients from the food. Proper chewing leads to improved digestion. So, take care of your teeth. If you are missing teeth, discuss this with your dentist. There may be some resources available to assist you in repair and replacement.

Taking care of your mouth includes gum health. Chronic gum disease can cause problems with your blood sugar. Regular dental exams will keep a check on your gum health.

Skincare – Think of your skin as a large band-aid. Your skin is the largest organ of your body. You must make every effort to protect your skin. Any break or wound makes you susceptible to infection. One of the side effects of diabetes is dry skin. Dry skin is more apt to have cracks, wounds, and sores. Take extra effort to keep your skin moisturized. Look for lotions or creams that do not dry the skin out. The best products to use are those formulated for people with diabetes. Use the products that work best for you.

The soap you use for bathing or showering determines what happens to your skin. A word about bathing. Prefer taking showers over baths because of exposure to heat and drying effects.

Foot care — Inspect your feet daily! Foot health is essential because you only get one pair. Varicose veins are problems with circulation in the legs. They can influence your feet. The feet are the farthest away from the heart, so blood must travel through impaired vessels. The problem worsens with aging. There is good circulation if there is hair on the toes. A five-step check can ensure that foot health is maintained.

1. Inspect your feet daily. Look at the bottoms, in between the toes, and at the tops of the feet and toes. You're checking for redness, blisters, skin breakdown, and all kind of wounds.

2. Search for corns or calluses. That means there is some uneven wear on your feet or poorly fitting shoes.

3. Limited mobility can prevent thorough examination. Use a hand mirror to look at the bottom of your feet. Or you can put the mirror on the floor and hold your foot above it.

4. It is important to check in between the toes. A fungal infection or athlete's foot can occur. Skin breaks between the toes can lead to infection.

5. Moisturize your feet every day after bathing, and it will decrease the risk of skin breaks and cracking because of dryness. Pay special attention to the heels. That area is more prone to dryness and cracking. Use lotion or cream on the soles and top of the feet but avoid using products between the

toes. Lotion or cream between the toes increases the risk of fungal infection.

Footcare

1. **Use an emery board to shorten your nails.** Using clippers or scissors can put you at risk of cutting the skin. Any skin break can lead to infection. With diabetes, there may be bad circulation. The proper way to file the nails is to file straight across. Avoid curving the nails because of the risk of developing ingrown toenails.

2. **Always wear some type of shoe.** Make sure you always have something on your feet, even if you're at the beach or if you're at a pool. Wearing slides are better than flip flops because the toe divider can irritate. If you have lost feeling in your feet, walking on hot sand can burn your feet. There can be objects in the sand too, that can hurt your feet.

3. **How to pick the right shoe**. A podiatrist can measure and fit you for the right shoe. If you don't see a podiatrist, take a sheet of paper, and stand on it. Have someone draw an outline of your foot while standing. Use this outline to choose your shoe. Compare the shoe outline with the bottom or sole of the shoe you want to buy. This is the time to buy shoes that are comfortable, flexible, breathable, and provide stability for standing and walking.

You only get one set of feet, so protect them. Diabetic or peripheral neuropathy is a complication of long-term diabetes. It can lead to loss of sensation to your feet. You could step on something and not realize it. **Storytime:** I have a friend who has a pool. She says she won't even go to a public pool because of the risk of developing an infection. She wears slides even though she has a personal pool. She said something can be in the bottom of the pool. Her words are, "I have to protect my feet."

It takes only one incident to cause a serious problem. You can end up with a wound that takes forever to heal. And if it doesn't heal, you can lose a toe, a foot, or a leg. I know that sounds gruesome, but that's the truth. I have seen too many times where people have been lax in protecting their feet and end up losing a limb.

Story time. This is one of the worst cases I've ever seen. My first patient of the day. This lady had severe burns on her feet and ankles. She said they were cold, so she put her feet by the heater. She did not have any sensation in her legs and feet. One of the first things that happens with neuropathy is cold feet. Because they cannot feel the temperature change, they risk burning themselves. So, I say, put on some socks, even two pair if you need them. Wrap your legs and feet in a blanket but whatever you do, do not put your feet by the heater.

Chapter 10: Sick Day Management

Be prepared for a sick day. Having diabetes puts you at risk for illness. Being older, in addition to diabetes, puts you at higher risk. The first sign you may notice is an increase in your blood sugar. Your body reacts to the illness first. When you notice the hyperglycemia (high blood sugar), drink 8 ounces of water every hour to remain hydrated. If you have a fever, use Tylenol.

A stomach virus or similar illness can occur suddenly. Start treating any vomiting and diarrhea immediately if it occurs. Fluid replacement is essential. Pedialyte may be a good fluid replacement but be careful of sugar content. Another choice is coconut water. Coconut water contains the electrolytes that you need to replace those fluids that are lost. But look at the label to get the one with the lowest sugar content. Here are some steps to take when you become ill.

- Take your medications as prescribed.

- Check your blood sugars more often when you are ill.

- Stay hydrated, drink something every hour.

- Soups and broths will provide nourishment.

- Eat small snacks to maintain blood sugar – fruit, Jello, saltines, peanut butter, yogurt.

- Use cold medicines made specifically for high blood pressure such as Coricidin HBP. Choose the one that has your symptoms listed.

- Recommend Robitussin DM or Delsym for dry cough. Mucinex DM is good for productive cough - to liquefy thick secretions.

- Be cautious with separate Tylenol when taking combination cold medicines. Many cold medicines contain Tylenol for reducing fever. It will be too easy to overdose on Tylenol.

- If taking liquid medicines, avoid those that contain sugar.

- For diarrhea –Use Imodium or Kaopectate

- Have a thermometer to check the temperature.

- Ginger ale is good to have for nausea. Have both diet and regular on hand.

Call your provider or go to Urgent Care or the emergency room if your condition worsens, blood sugars are higher than 300, and not going down. Other red flags warrant immediate attention – prolonged diarrhea, lasting more than 6 hours or more than five incidents, and repeated vomiting. These incidents are dangerous because they can cause a chemical imbalance in your body.

Heat exposure and injury

Being out in the heat for long periods puts you at risk for heat injury. This is especially true for those over the age of 50. The danger is dehydration plus loss of vital minerals, especially salt. So, you go from dehydration to heat injury, to heat stroke. And that's the continuum if you don't take in enough fluids.

The problem is that as you get older, you tend not to drink as much fluid. The general statement I hear is "I'm not thirsty". The key to avoiding dehydration is to drink fluids, especially water, regularly throughout the day. When you make it a habit to drink 8 – 16 ounces every 1-2 hours, you will remain hydrated. Your body will start triggering the thirst components.

Another complaint I hear is drinking more will cause more trips to the bathroom. Think of all the waste products and toxins being removed every time you go to the bathroom. Drinking fluids flush out your system.

The benefits of increased water intake:

- Good hydration thins out the blood; keeps your blood flowing.

- Improves muscle health and prevents acid buildup in muscle cells.

- Skin will be clearer with toxins and debris removed from your body

- Clarity of thinking - Removal of toxins will improve mental processes.

- Improved digestion – Digestive juices flow and break down food

- Decrease hunger – feel fuller when drinking water before meals.

- Decreased joint and back pain – increased water fills the cushions between joints and the spinal column

- Improve kidney health – water will flush out the kidneys to improve their function.

- Improve stamina with exercise – muscle function improves when well hydrated.

Chapter 11: Checkups and Prevention

Regular primary care visits should be every 3-6 months, depending on your blood sugar readings and other labs. Sometimes we stay focused on diabetes and neglect the other parts of our body. Some tests are recommended, especially over the age of 50.

- Colonoscopy – starting at the age of 45 to screen for colon cancer.

- Mammogram – to be done annually.

- Pap smear and vaginal exam – to be done annually

- Bone density test – to screen for osteoporosis. Start at 50 years old or at menopause, whichever comes first

- Chest x-ray – annually if you're a smoker.

- Aortic ultrasound – at age 65 if smoker. Checking for aneurysm

- Prostate exam for men. Digital rectal exam and prostate specific antigen (PSA) blood test should be part of annual exam. I strongly recommend digital rectal exam. PSA can give you a false negative.

Vaccines

These are important because of being over 50 years old and having diabetes. These put you at high risk for disease.

- Flu vaccine – once a year

- Pneumonia vaccine – If given after 65 years old, it does not need to be repeated. If taken before 65 and high risk, it may need to repeat after the age of 65. Check with your provider about the types of pneumonia vaccines available.

- COVID vaccine and booster

- Tdap – tetanus once every ten years

- Shingles vaccine – series of 2 injections after the age of 50

- Hepatitis B vaccine – recommended for type 2 diabetes adults younger than 60. Series of 3 vaccines.

- Other vaccines may be recommended for overseas travel.

Chapter 12: Heart Disease and Diabetes

Heart disease is a common complication among people with diabetes. Type 2 diabetes does not exist alone. It is usually accompanied by high blood pressure and high cholesterol. Uncontrolled blood pressure over a period can cause abnormalities in the heart. The increased pressure can lead to heart enlargement.

The most prevalent time for heart disease to present itself in women is after menopause. Loss of naturally occurring estrogen increases the risk of heart disease.

Storytime – This occurred with one lady I knew – we'll call her Linda. She told someone at work that she was having trouble breathing. But Linda decided to go home after work. (She worked for a hospital). She told her mother that she just didn't feel well when she got home.　Linda went to her room to get ready for bed. After a while, Linda's daughter called her grandmother to say that she could not reach her mother by phone.

The grandmother went to check on Linda. She found Linda slumped over in a chair. EMS was unable to revive Linda, and she was pronounced dead. Linda was 60 years old, without any health problems, and worked every day.

Heart disease and heart attacks in women have different presentations than in men. Heart disease is commonly referred to as coronary artery disease (CAD). This is characterized by abnormal cholesterol. This abnormal cholesterol is characterized by high levels of LDL (bad)lipoprotein and low HDL (good) lipoprotein. The high LDL can cause fatty substances known as plaque build-up in the coronary arteries. This build-up limits the amount of blood getting to the heart. Arteries carry blood from the heart to vital parts such as the heart, lungs, kidney, and brain. Uncontrolled diabetes is elevated blood sugar. This uncontrolled blood sugar has large glucose (sugar) molecules in the circulation. High glucose causes the blood to be too thick and more prone to clotting.

Another problem with high glucose is its damage to the small vessels in the body – the eye, the kidney, and the heart. To focus on the heart – small vessel damage is especially bad in women because the vessels tend to be smaller. Limited blood flow to the heart means no oxygen can get to that part of the heart muscle and can lead to muscle damage.

The most common complaint is unexplained fatigue. This is a new development. The fatigue comes from a decrease in oxygen to the body. If you have trouble walking to the mailbox, something you have always done. That is a new symptom. Another symptom is sleep disruption or unable to sleep. 48% of these 500 women surveyed said they had trouble sleeping. Chest pain is not a typical sign of a heart attack in women. The biggest complaint they have is fatigue and shortness of breath. These symptoms can be present for some time before a heart attack happens.

What causes a Heart Attack?
A previous discussion explained cholesterol levels and uncontrolled blood sugar. A heart attack is when a blood clot or a piece of plaque breaks off and blocks an artery. That blocked artery prevents blood flow and oxygen from getting to that part of the heart. That's what causes the pain.

Some of the common symptoms that you will find are:

1. Nausea
2. Vomiting
3. Indigestion
4. Fatigue
5. Lightheadedness
6. Pain in the neck, jaw, back, throat

These are typical symptoms that women feel. That is why these symptoms get ignored or overlooked.

Storytime: Several years ago, I had an episode of severe indigestion. Because of my history of ulcers, I ignored it. So, I started drinking more water, thinking that it was something I had eaten and needed to dilute it. The next morning, the pain returned after I started exercising. That was my red flag. I called a colleague who worked in cardiology and saw me immediately. Based on my symptoms, the cardiologist did a heart cath. Thank God everything was clear. But there are too many instances where women have ignored the symptoms and had a massive heart attack.

If you have a family history of heart disease, especially if you had heart problems before the age of 50, you need an evaluation. Don't let them ignore your complaints. You need to get checked out. Women's anatomy is different from men. Our vessels are smaller. So, a regular stress test may not detect abnormalities in a woman. Suggest a nuclear stress test because it can visualize the smaller vessels. I recommend going to your provider if you are having symptoms. It's best to know that everything is clear early rather than having to go for emergency testing and surgery.

Chapter 13: Menopause and Diabetes

Menopause is a normal part of life. It is part of the natural aging process. If you had a hysterectomy and ovaries removed before age 50, that was surgical menopause. You're going from childbearing to non-childbearing. You're going from one stage to another, and that's a transition. And sometimes, that transition can be kind of rocky. Some women have a harder time with menopause than others.

Menopause has 3 phases.

- Perimenopause – Irregular periods occur. This stage can occur up to 10 years before menopause. Hot flashes and night sweats start to occur in the 40s. This is probably due to a decrease in progesterone levels. You may notice problems with sleep.

- Menopause - No period for one full year.

- Post menopause – After the full transition.

The goal is for you to feel normal. You will develop a new normal.

Symptoms of menopause:
- Hot flashes and night sweats

- Breast tenderness

- Heavier and unpredictable periods – due to the diminishing levels of estrogen in the body

- Mood swings – can experience depression and/or anxiety.

- Sleep disturbances – related to the fluctuating estrogen levels and increased cortisol production.

- Migraine – may lessen if estrogen triggers them.

- Aches and pains – related to the aging process and diminished estrogen. It takes longer to recover from strenuous exercise sessions.

- Vaginal dryness and atrophy – related to low estrogen and the effect of diabetes.

- Bone loss – more prone to osteopenia or osteoporosis because of low estrogen. Regular, routine weight-bearing exercise can counteract this effect.

- Increased cardiovascular disease risk – loss of estrogen lead to decreased cardio protection.

To be proactive, lower the LDL cholesterol with medication and raise the HDL by routine exercise. Remember 150 – 200 minutes per week exercise is recommended. This activity will give you a double benefit by strengthening your bones too. If you are new to exercise or have not exercised in some time, it is best to do short, mild to moderate intensity types of exercises. Lack of estrogen affects your ability to recover from exercise. Vigorous activity may require a rest day for full recovery.

Chapter 14: Be Your Own Advocate

All clients with diabetes need to know how to advocate for themselves. Advocacy means getting support from another person to help you stand up for your rights. In this case, you, the patient, must be your own advocate. Many times, people go to the provider visits alone, and there is no one else there to speak up for them. So, you need to know how to speak up for yourself.

I want to provide you with the information and tools you need to use for your provider visits. The day is over when you, the patient, sit and listen to the provider give directions. The key in today's provider climate is shared decision-making and client-centered care. The office visit should be a discussion between the provider and the patient. The benefit of shared decision-making is encouraging clients to have a strong voice in their care. When the provider participates, it shows respect for the client and their values. Clients with diabetes who learn how to advocate often benefit from getting a better understanding of their health and learning all they can about diabetes. The patient knows their body and how they are feeling Clients with diabetes need to be honest with their provider about how they feel. This is not the time to be shy or reluctant to tell your provider about your symptoms. The best thing you can do is start writing down what symptoms you are experiencing and when they occur. Get into the habit of writing notes down in a designated notebook or your phone. That way, you have the notes to remind you what you wanted to discuss during your visit. Discussing the concerns with the provider helps to improve your visit and gives insight to your provider.

If your provider has advised you to check your blood sugar, write it down. It is helpful to write down the time and what you ate too. This can provide information on what treatment would be best for you.

I recommend getting a home blood pressure cuff. Most people with diabetes have high blood pressure, too. It would be helpful to check your blood pressure at least once daily and write it down too. Take your readings to your visit so your provider can see how your numbers are running at home. Some people have high blood pressure readings at the office. So, it is good to have the home readings for comparison.

Are you taking your medications as prescribed? You, the patient, need to be honest with the provider about prescribed medications. Some patients don't like taking pills, so they don't take them as ordered. There may be times that you, the patient, go to the pharmacy for medications and cannot afford the medicine. You need to let the provider know that you are not taking the medicines. And be honest in telling them why. Let them know you don't remember to take your medications. Or if you cannot afford a medicine, let them know. They may have samples or prescription drug programs available to make the medicines more affordable.

It is especially important to let the provider know if you had an allergic reaction to a medicine. Tell them what the reaction was and when it occurred. That way, they can record it in your chart. Also, let your pharmacist know, too. That will prevent any problems with medication interactions. This is another form of advocacy.

Understand Your Lab Results – Don't be afraid to ask

Another form of advocacy is asking for an explanation of the lab results. Clients with diabetes need to understand their results. The most important areas to focus on are chemistry, lipid panel, A1C, and blood count. In chemistry, the most important tests are glucose, potassium, kidney function, and liver function. Ask the provider to explain the lab results in easy-to-understand terms. If the provider does not have time to review the labs, ask if the nurse can review them and answer any questions. Ask for a copy of the labs to take home. Keep all lab results for comparison - to see how the labs are trending. That means to see if there's any change from the previous labs. Find out when you need to follow up for any abnormal labs. Ask if a referral to a specialist is needed. Once you know what the tests mean, you will be more diligent in self-care to improve your readings. The main benefit of advocacy is to get the best care possible. The goal of therapy is to prevent or control diabetes, avoid preventable complications and hospitalizations. The desired result of advocacy is having the best treatment plan possible.

Chapter 15: Putting It All Together

This book contains a lot of information. It is a compilation of much research and years of experience in working with people. Now comes the implementation. How are you going to apply this information into your life? My recommendation is a stepped approach, take it one part at a time.

- Adopt a growth mindset – You have the ability to change

- Make time – Set aside time to plan

- Take action – don't get stuck in analyzing, take action on one thing

- Change is hard – Understand that you are changing lifelong habits. That is hard.

- Be reasonable and realistic about what you can do.

- Focus on the process, not the outcome

Now to choose your goals. What do you want to work on first? Usually when you start with one healthy change, others will automatically follow. The key is consistency.

- Set your goal

- What skills do you need to reach your goal

- How do you plan, prioritize, and prepare

- How do you make time for this skill

- How are you going to keep track of your progress.

Let's set an example. Let's say you have not been walking and you are going to start walking 5 days a week.

Plan: Where are you going to walk? Map out a safe and easy route. Do you have the right equipment? Get some good walking shoes to prevent any foot problems.

Prioritize: What time of day are you going to walk? You want to set a plan that has the least number of obstacles or problems.

Plan: Prepare by setting your clothes out the night before. Mark off on your calendar or phone each day you go for a walk. Log how long you walked or how far.

Review your progress at the end of you 5 days. How did you do? How do you feel? How did your blood sugar do?

This book provides tools and information to get you started.

Give yourself some grace. Change will not occur overnight. The problems did not happen overnight. This change happens gradually over time. Lifestyle behavior change is developing a new lifestyle. You have decided to have a makeover, one small change at a time.

Everything is not for everybody. Everybody's body is different. Everybody's preferences are different. Don't fall into the trap of comparing yourself to someone else. Determine what your journey is going to be. It's never too late to make a change for your health. You are never too old to make a difference.

Chapter 16: Summary

Type 2 diabetes is a chronic disease that comes from lifestyle habits and family history. Diabetes is at pandemic levels in the United States. 37.3 million people in the US have diabetes.

The problem that I have identified there is a lack of understanding of the diabetes education. The way 3rd party payors cover diabetes education is at time of diagnosis is around 10 hours – 9 of those hours are for group training.

I believe that close follow up is needed to provide training, education, and support to change these longstanding lifestyle habits. The best results come when the client is motivated to change, willing to learn about the disease, take the information they learn and implement it. The client decides what action or what changes they are willing do. You are that client.

"Our lifestyle choices, driven by our behavior, account for over half of the risk of early death. What we do every single day matters. Just like a new skill, good health requires work. That work is personal, and it looks a bit different for everyone, but effort is needed." Dr. Mark Hyman

Use the gift offered at the beginning of the book to set up your program. Contact me when you are ready to get started.